How You Look and How You Feel.
Personal Transformation.

I0967723

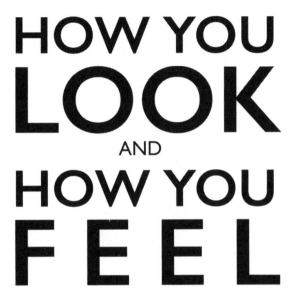

HOW YOU
LOOK
AND
HOW YOU
FEEL

Personal Transformation

Van Harden

XULON PRESS

Xulon Press
2301 Lucien Way #415
Maitland, FL 32751
407.339.4217
www.xulonpress.com

© 2018 by Van Harden

All rights reserved solely by the author. The author guarantees all contents are original and do not infringe upon the legal rights of any other person or work. No part of this book may be reproduced in any form without the permission of the author. The views expressed in this book are not necessarily those of the publisher.

Printed in the United States of America.

ISBN-13: 978-1-54564-557-4

Table of Contents

Chapter One

The Introduction

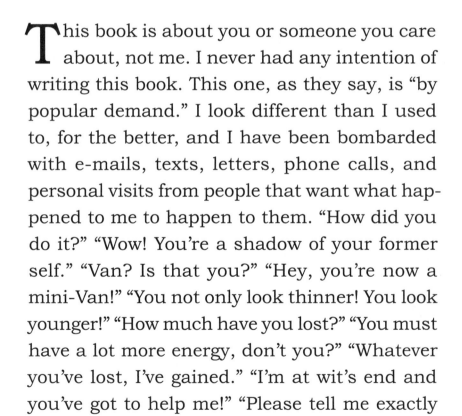

This book is about you or someone you care about, not me. I never had any intention of writing this book. This one, as they say, is "by popular demand." I look different than I used to, for the better, and I have been bombarded with e-mails, texts, letters, phone calls, and personal visits from people that want what happened to me to happen to them. "How did you do it?" "Wow! You're a shadow of your former self." "Van? Is that you?" "Hey, you're now a mini-Van!" "You not only look thinner! You look younger!" "How much have you lost?" "You must have a lot more energy, don't you?" "Whatever you've lost, I've gained." "I'm at wit's end and you've got to help me!" "Please tell me exactly what you have done." "Have you written about this anywhere? Because I've got to read it."

I've heard all these things and more lately. Yes, I've worked on losing weight, and yes it has been successful, but I had no idea the kind of response it would bring from others, not just in compliments, but in the revealing of personal desperation by many. I am constantly having to re-tell the story because of so many people asking. So, it's time to write it out and apparently a wonderful opportunity to help people, or at least try. Not that I have all the answers, since everyone is different. But many are asking in much more than an inquisitive way. Many are clearly hurting, desperate to change, and even depressed about how they look and how they feel. Frankly, I never dreamed I would be in a position like this. In fact, I was asked to be the keynote speaker for a health conference a while back. I told them all that if you would have told me the year before that I would be asked to be a keynote speaker at a health conference, I would have said, "Ya, right, and next you're gonna tell me the Cubs will win the World Series, or that Donald Trump will become President!"

At my peak, I had lost a hundred-and-three pounds. It stays fairly steady around a hundred now. I really do not feel like an expert at any of this. All I can tell you is where I was, what happened, what action I took, and the results. I lost seventy pounds in the first eight months. Many of you will probably think that no one should lose that much weight that quickly, and that those are the kinds of "diets" in which a person gains all the weight back, usually plus more. That's probably true more often than not, but I truly believe I found a healthy way around that, at least for me.

As a disclaimer, before you decide you'd like to dive into something like this, there is something I feel is important to say. My thought is that people think about themselves far too much and far too often and that includes me. As one who is guilty of this, I totally understand why. This is the only world in which we've ever lived. We only get one body and none of us got to make a custom order. Then we often don't treat it very well when we get it. The human default mindset seems to be, "How can I get what I want to be happy?" Much of that happiness seems to be based on how you look and how you feel.

Yes, it pleases me that I weigh less. Yes, it pleases me that I get so many compliments about how I look. I guess deep down we all desire that, but when it happens, even though it brings happiness, it doesn't necessarily bring true joy. I've often been amazed at some of the truly beautiful Hollywood type people that have committed suicide. The immediate thought is how that could possibly happen when they were so rich and looked so terrific, as though those were the yardsticks of happiness.

I know many people that are basing their pending happiness on certain things happening. They are sure they will be happy if only this or that happens. Many people die waiting. That's sad. It's come to my attention, through this experience, that personal appearance is one of those things.

I hope this book will be useful to those of you seeking help. But as many of you know all too well, pounds come and go. My experience may bring you some success and happiness. I will be honored indeed if that happens. But you need Someone much bigger than Van Harden for you to receive true joy, no matter how you look or how you feel physically.

There. I got that off my chest. Now we may proceed with how you look and how you feel.

Get out your high-light marker and get ready to mark the things that seem to especially pertain to you. Let's dig in!

Chapter Two

The Situation

I wasn't happy with the way I looked. I wasn't happy with the way I felt. I was tired most of the time. In fact, I caught myself falling asleep at my desk in the afternoon during my administrative duties at work. I was thinking…oh no! Sleep apnea! It was an ego blow, when I woke up on my own and realized what had happened. Even worse was when someone would come to see me in my office and be awkwardly caught by surprise at my state, and not know what to say or do. Usually I woke up, but I wonder how many people did that, were embarrassed, and left quickly, and I just didn't know it.

As far as eating was concerned, I loved to do it and there were very few things I didn't like to eat. The things I liked best were the ones that were worst for me. Sound familiar? Plus, eating can be such a mind game. I actually remember a few times being frustrated that I was full because I wanted to eat some more!

I have been a radio broadcaster since 1971 and for about thirty two years of that time, I have been getting up at three in the morning to host a morning show on WHO Radio in Des Moines. It's never easy to get up at that time of day, but it kept getting harder...and harder...... and harder, to the point at which I didn't know how much longer I could keep doing it. When I got a cold it would last longer than normal and breathing became more and more difficult. One time, in particular, I actually thought I was dying and went to the emergency room of a hospital, which is totally unlike me. That's how bad it was. It was a move of desperation. I was given some antibiotics and over a long period of time I slowly felt better, even though I wasn't.

After the episodes of falling asleep at my desk, the difficulties of getting up in the morning, and extended colds and breathing problems, I came to the conclusion there had to be some-thing seriously wrong with me. Again, I was convinced I was dying. That's how I looked, and that's how I felt. I uncharacteristically decided

I needed a doctor, not so much to cure me, but to find out how it was that I was going to die, and start making preparations for whatever time was left. I had no family doctor and no idea who to call. I remembered an orthopedic surgeon I had interviewed on the air. He and I were about the same age and really hit it off. I knew I didn't need an orthopedic surgeon, but I did need his advice and connections.

I called him, told him my situation, and that I didn't know what to do. Just like a Jerry Seinfeld routine, he said, "Oh, ya gotta see my doctor! He's the best!". I think Jerry's point was that nobody ever says his or her doctor is the worst. Anyway, he said his guy was an internist and that if I started at a lower level than that, they'd keep passing me up the chain till I got to someone like him and that would take a lot of time and effort. He said he didn't know whether his guy would even take on a new patient, since he was highly respected, successful and sought-after. He called me back later that day and said, "I got you in! Just call his office and make an appointment." I did.

Oddly enough, before all this, I had been helping the Governor's office and Hy-Vee grocery stores in promoting the "Iowa Healthiest State" initiative, encouraging people to eat right and exercise. What a hypocrite! I was far from being a role model. That's how all this started, but before I tell you what happened next, I'm going to tell you the final results so you don't get a papercut turning to the back of the book.

I have lost a hundred pounds. I no longer fall asleep at my desk. I very seldom have colds, and the one I had lasted only a few days rather than weeks or months. My breathing is completely normal. My cholesterol and blood pressure are in check. But most amazingly to me, I look different. Some of my friends I hadn't seen for a while had to do double takes. I'm told I look ten years younger. I was asked to do a cameo appearance at the local playhouse. The bit was that I would be on stage with the rest of the cast in their medieval costuming and me in armor with a helmet disguising my true identity. Then, halfway through the show, the lead actor would come over, remove my helmet, and the crowd would be totally surprised and thrilled that their local, long-time radio and TV personality, Van Harden, was revealed and great joy, laughing and applause would ensue!

This was right after I had lost all the weight and looked different. There was only a lukewarm response, and as it turned out, people didn't know it was me! I didn't look like the old Van. I looked like Mini-Van and the audience had never seen him before. Also, I had to have my driver's license photo retaken since I no longer looked like the one I was carrying and it caused some real problems, once at the airport!

So, there is the situation and the results. Now, here is the part everybody asks me about......"What did you do?!"

Chapter Three

The Doctor's Office

Appointment day came and I headed to the doctor's office. I checked in at the desk and they handed me an Etch-a-Sketch. At least that's what it looked like. But it was an electronic registration system on which you answered questions with a stylus. You've probably done it yourself. I wasn't wild about it but it has actually saved me a lot of time and questioning with return visits and with other specialists, and believe me, I'd be seeing a lot of them! Younger folks were doing fine with theirs. Older people weren't. I kinda wanted to stick around to see if anybody would turn theirs upside down and shake it to erase it.

My name was called and the doctor's assistant escorted me down the hall to the scale. I weighed in. She noted the weight, wrote it down, said "Thank you" without saying anything else except to follow her down the hall. You see, that's the difference between her profession and mine. My inclination as a smart aleck radio host, when seeing a number that large, would have been to say something like, "Please sir, only one person on the scale at a time!" She took me to the exam room, asked some questions, took my vitals and said the doctor would be right in. And he was.

He was a very pleasant guy, but got right down to business as he asked my reason for being there. I said, "Well, you can see on the chart my age. I get up every weekday morning at three o'clock. I often put in twelve or thirteen hour workdays, and I know I'm overweight. If anybody has the right to be tired, it's probably me, but I need to know if there's something else going on that I should know about."

He gave me a quick check, but scheduled many tests from many specialists. These tests did not miss one inch of the human anatomy, inside or out. I spent the next month leaving work frequently after I got off the air for these tests. Some were tolerable. Some were extremely unpleasant. They were very time consuming. I considered not going to some of them, but I did them all.

Meanwhile before leaving the room with the original doctor, he did an extensive interview, asking me many questions. In my work, I am usually the one doing the interviewing and asking the questions, so this was odd for me. He asked about my sleeping, eating, physical activity, lifestyle, work and emotional state.

It is here that we get to the heart of the reason you may have wanted to read this book. Here is part of the conversation.

Dr.... What do you have for breakfast?

Van.... I don't have breakfast.

Dr.... Why not?

Van.... I'm on the radio at that time.

Dr.... What do you have for lunch?

Van.... (sheepishly) Well, most of the time I don't have lunch.

Dr.... Why not?

Van... I'm just so busy. I never stop and I seldom even think about it.

Dr.... So, if you don't eat breakfast and you don't eat lunch, when DO you eat?

Van.... When I get home at five......and at six...... and at seven.

He slapped his forehead, rolled his chair over to his little desk, got out a sheet of paper and started writing.

Dr.... OK, for the next month, here's exactly what you're gonna be eating. If you have any complaints about this, you'll have to talk to my wife, because this is what she's got me on. It's not very complicated. For breakfast, which you'll have to start eating right after you get off the air at nine am, you'll have a bowl of steel cut oatmeal with walnuts and raisins. For lunch, you'll have one six ounce cup of yogurt. For dinner have a boneless, skinless chicken breast or fish with a vegetable. If you want a dessert, have some fruit. Drink water. That's it!

Van.... That's it?

Dr.... That's it. And I'm giving you three prescription drugs addressing things appropriate for you.

He explained what they were and why he was prescribing them. I could live with the prescribed food menu, but I took exception to the drugs. I've prided myself in not taking drugs of any kind, and I told him so. I even knew of the side effects and problems some people have had from them. "I came in here today drug-free and I intend to go out the same way, if not today, then soon," I told him.

On the other hand, it was me, and no one else, that came to him with the problem, so I decided I should do what he said with an understanding that I had two clear goals. #1 to get rid of the drugs. And #2 to get rid of him! He laughed hard when I said that, and said "I totally get that and those are worthy goals." He's been a close personal friend ever since.

He asked me to make an appointment for one month later. I scheduled it, then left, and made two stops...the office supply store and the grocery store.

At the office supply place, I bought a 7 by 4 ½ inch notebook. At the grocery store, I bought walnuts, raisins, a box with ten pouches of steel cut oatmeal, ten cups of yogurt in a variety of flavors, boneless, skinless chicken breasts, and from the produce department, broccoli, asparagus, fresh blueberries and strawberries. So the new way of eating began, and I had a notepad to write down what I ate every day. I guess that's called personal accountability. Occasionally when I didn't do as well as I wanted, I thought about just not writing down something I ate, but I thought only a knuckle head would cheat on himself. After all, I was the only one that was going to be seeing my food diary.

One thing I've noticed is that when people end diets, they gain weight. There's a way around that. Don't go on a diet. Just change the way you eat permanently so there's no diet to end. I even remember a time when I and others would celebrate reaching a goal of a diet by going out to eat! Wow! Seriously, how dumb are we?

I've never been a smoker, but I have had friends and loved ones that were. I've had tremendous admiration for them when they decided they had enough and were going to completely quit all at once. I decided I would have to have that same commitment and mindset in my situation. No sneaking foods, drinks or snacks! Absolutely not! I said seriously, to myself, "Van, do you really want this or not? Because if you're not completely committed to this, you're gonna fail!" So, like an alcoholic making the life changing commitment, I made the commitment to absolutely be on this plan in such a way that it wasn't really even a plan anymore, but a way of life.....forever.

One last thing about that original meeting with the doctor. I told him honestly I hated exercising, knowing full well he was going to get around to that topic eventually. He smiled and said, "Yes, a lot of my patients do. All I'm going to ask is that you walk for thirty minutes five days a week." I said okay, wondering how many patients tell him okay on food and exercise, then never do it or try it, only to give up.

The grueling, time consuming, emotionally draining month of tests went by and I'll save you the details, even though you sadists might like to hear about my colonoscopy, at which I refused sedation. Remember I mentioned I don't want to be on drugs?. Well, most people probably should take the drugs before a colonoscopy, but I actually did just fine without them and I got to watch the whole procedure on a big screen, high definition TV monitor, ask questions, learn a lot from the doctor and he even asked me a few radio questions during the procedure. Plus, I didn't need a driver to get home, even though I had one, and I wasn't loopy that afternoon. In fact when I got home, I mowed my yard. If you have a medical background you're probably cringing. Come to think of it, you may be cringing even without a medical background. I'm not recommending a colonoscopy without the drug regimen they usually put you through before it, but I did it without.

Some of you might have been through what I thought was the most embarrassing part of the procedure after it was over. I never really envisioned being alone in a room with an attractive young nurse urging me to release gas. In fact, don't most women encourage exactly the opposite? But when I didn't produce, she started pushing on my stomach to help the process along. Then, when it finally happened, I got huge congratulations, kinda like when you were potty training your kids and it finally happened. Anyway, I said I'd spare you the details, but you did get a few.

So, now, after all those medical visits it was time to focus on the menu and the exercise.

Chapter Four

The Ball's in Your Court

The next morning after that first doctor's visit, I started the food plan. It was odd to eat at all in the morning, especially oatmeal with walnuts and raisins, but I did it at nine am and have done so every morning since then. On page one of my notebook, I wrote it down.

At noon, I had one of my yogurts and I wrote that down too. By the way, when I would leave for work each morning, I would grab a yogurt, without looking at the flavor, and take it to work. After I did this for a few days, I realized it really seemed rather pathetic that one of the big thrills of my day came at noon, opening the refrigerator door and being surprised by what flavor I got that day, but it's been kinda fun.

For dinner, I had a boneless, skinless chicken breast, broccoli, and blueberries, all of which I wrote down as well. The doctor had never said a thing about writing down what I ate, but I thought it would be a good idea not only for my own records, but to hold myself accountable for what I ate. Even though the doctor had said that I should eat the food he recommended for the next month, I did not stop after that. I kept to that food routine and I wrote it all down. It's not a diet, it's a way of life and I intend to do it till I die.

The doctor had passed me the ball. It was in my court. It was either play offense or sit on the bench and snack. I knew that only one person in the world would ever make this happen. It wasn't the doctor, it wasn't a personal trainer, a family member, an accountability group, or a friend. Yes, there was only one person that could make this happen, and I knew that person very, very well. Many people use many different methods to lose weight and get healthier. Everyone's different and what's right for one person may not be right for another. The only thing I can tell you is my own experience. In my case it had to be me, myself, and I with prayer and divine intervention in order for it to work.

Chapter Five

The First Follow-Up

Asrequested, I went back in a month for a check-up. I had already lost enough weight that it was noticeable, plus as I remembered from before, they weigh you before you see the doctor each time you visit. The doctor looked at me and looked at the charts and was all smiles. That was quite a contrast to the way he looked on that first appointment. He had actually looked depressed. Back then I remember thinking it must be pretty bad if your doctor looks depressed. Shouldn't I be the one that was depressed?

"What have you been doing?" he asked.

I said, "What do you mean, what have I been doing? You've sent me to every specialist in town and I've had every test in the book."

He laughed and said, "Ya, I got all the test results, but how are you losing weight?"

"Well, Doc," I said, "I could show you my little book of exactly what I have eaten and exactly what exercise I have been doing every day, but I'm sure that would be boring to you."

"Absolutely not!" he said. "Let me see that book!" He scooted his chair over to the little desk and went through every word of every page, all the while uttering, "This is amazing. This is amazing. You are my rock star patient! Do you know how many people come through my door on a regular basis, much like you, and ask for help? I tell them pretty much the same thing I told you, but you are one of the few that is actually doing it! You are a real morale boost to me. You make this all worth it. You are to be congratulated!" He wasn't depressed this time. He was happy. And it made me happy to see him so happy!

I thanked him but reminded him that I was the one that came to him for help, and that it would seem rather foolish to reject the very help that I sought. Plus, I reminded him again, "I still want to get rid of these prescriptions and I still want to get rid of you." He laughed harder this time than he did the first time. Then he said he wanted me to come back again in another month.

I didn't laugh and said, "Again?"

"Yes," he said. "I just have a hard time believing you can keep this up. I want to track it."

So, much to my dismay, I booked another appointment, went in, and having lost even more weight, he opened the door to the exam room and said, "Nurses, come see this guy!" Again, I was happy for him, but a bit embarrassed for myself.

I was amazed that all this was happening. People were treating me differently, even though I was the same guy. I was being successful at something I knew a lot of other people wanted for themselves.

Two quick words of advice….if you do indeed have success, be ready for how other people respond to it and don't ever, ever get cocky about it or take it for granted. It could change in a few moments if you're not thankful and careful. Instead of basking in glory, ask yourself how you might use your success to help others.

Chapter Six

The Exercise

Some people love exercise. They'll pay a lot of money for personal trainers, fitness club memberships, exercise equipment, and more. If you're one of those, you're probably way ahead of the game in this "How you look and how you feel" thing.

I am not one of those people, and I imagine that this chapter is going to be more for people like me than you physical movers-and-shakers but it's interesting how many of the latter have asked me for advice. Even they have weight and fitness challenges. By the way, I'll never forget the time I was given a tour of a fitness center. I noticed that some people were taking the elevator up to the second floor to use the stair-step machines.

Clearly a lot of this entire experience of looking better and feeling better is a mind game. Since so many people have asked me to share what I'm doing, I hope this book will help you with whatever mind game might help you. Not only is everyone's body different, everyone's mind is different too. What works for one person may not work for you. That's why I emphasize that this book is by no means an end-all answer to the way you look and feel. However, the very fact that you've picked it up to read it indicates you are part-way there! You want to look good and feel good and you're willing to listen to ideas. If my ideas don't sound like something for you, maybe they will trip other ideas that will! I'm only an expert on what worked for me. That's what I've been asked to share and that's what I'm doing. Who knows? Maybe you'll be helping others with your own story before long!

Just like the doctor's advice with the menu of food and prescriptions, I again figured that if I was going to ask for help, I'd be stupid not to at least try the doctor's suggestion in regard to exercise. So I walked. I had been fairly sedentary, but I knew if I continued to do what I'd already done, I'd continue to get what I'd already got. That may be grammatically incorrect, but it's powerful. I'm sure you get the point. A similar thought that you frequently hear is that the definition of insanity is doing the same thing over and over, and expecting a different result. That's what I'd done. Is that what you're doing?

Walking is probably not that big of a deal for many people, especially you jocks. But I just had not been interested. The doc said do a half hour a day, so the day after that first doctor's appointment, when I got home from work, I walked. I live in the small town where I was raised, and so I walked around town.

I ran into a couple of problems right away. Since I'm fairly well known in the community, either as the guy on the radio or the hometown kid that used to mow everyone's yard, people would stop their cars as I was walking and yell, "Hey Van! Wanna ride?" My town is like Mayberry in the Andy Griffith show, and I wouldn't have it any other way, but I had to explain to these people that I was doing this as much for my doctor as I was for me.

The second problem was that people frequently wanted to stop me to talk. As anyone from a small town knows, there's a lot to talk about. Again, that's part of what makes the community so special, but I could see that this half-hour walking thing was not going to work out. Just like in a car, when you start and stop, you don't get very good mileage.

Other than that, the half hour of walking was not as bad as I thought it was going to be. Every house and building I walked by brought back memories of people, families and events from my childhood and beyond. Not only was that nostalgic and stimulating, it took my mind off the fact that I was walking. So I encourage you, if you have to walk, or want to, get creative about walking places that will stimulate your mind or interest you while you're also getting some exercise.

After being stopped so many times for "a ride" or conversation, I walked to the high school, which like many others, has a tartan track. I walked around four times, which is a mile, and I actually enjoyed it. So, I started going there every day. After doing it for a few days, I remember thinking, "This isn't so bad. Maybe I could do two miles." So I started walking around the track eight times instead of four.

Then I got into variations of the walk. Sometimes I would try walking as fast as I could and timed myself to try to beat my previous record. I never ran, or even jogged. I've had too many friends and acquaintances that have either sore knees, or have even had knee-replacement surgery. I didn't want to solve one problem while causing another.

One day, I noticed that behind some hurdles sitting next to the track, there were some sandbags used at their base so they didn't get knocked over. On my second lap that day, I picked up one of the sandbags and carried it around the track as I walked. On the next lap, I picked up another one and carried two of them. It was just an off-the-cuff, crazy, spontaneous thing, but I had a certain sense of pride when I was done. It also helped that nobody saw me do it!

When I was telling one of my co-workers about my walking, I mentioned that I hoped my body wasn't getting used to it, thus reducing its effectiveness. She said, "You ought to try walking backwards. You would be using an entirely different set of muscles." That made sense to me so I tried it that evening. I did three quarters of a lap and had a hard time with it. I kept going faster and faster and clearly would have fallen down if I hadn't stopped occasionally. I found it to be disorienting. I actually got somewhat dizzy. I now understand why God put the long part of our feet in front and not in the back! I finished the lap, have never done it since, and have no desire to do so again.

Every time I walked around that track, I looked at the stadium seating. I had flashbacks of the football, basketball and track practices when the coach would have us run up and down stairs until we were exhausted. So, the next time I went to the track I walked the stairs instead of the track. As heavy as I was, I wondered if I might be inviting a heart attack, so I was extremely careful about how many steps I did and how it made me feel. The first time I did fifty stairs, then added to that a bit at a time. Then it was a hundred. Then it was a thousand. Then it was twenty-five hundred. As I lost weight, it got easier to do since I didn't have as much weight to lift up the stairs. I only do this occasionally now, alternating with walking and other things I'll mention in the next chapter.

As much as I loved the track, I started getting bored with the scenery. It never changed. I really liked the softer walking surface the track provided, and it dawned on me that other schools had similar tracks. To make a long story short, I have gone to over thirty-five high school and college tracks in my area and walked eight laps on each. I keep driving further and further away from my home to do this, but the uniqueness of each one turned out to be fun, fascinating, and mind-stimulating. And it's made for some great radio stories. Guess what I don't even think about while I'm doing it? Walking!

Old habits and mind games die hard. I found myself driving to the closest possible parking spots at these stadiums so I didn't have to walk so far to the track to do my walking. What a dope!

I've only been kicked off of one track. The guy mowing the football field asked if I had the key to the gate, since he was going to lock up. I said no and he told me I had to go. I had only done three laps at the time, so I drove to another school and did the other five laps there. Most of these schools are fairly inviting about letting people walk on their tracks. Several even have signs that say "Welcome walkers". And that's the way it should be. Your tax dollars are helping pay for many of them. Plus schools are into teaching and they ought to be teaching good health, not just to the students but to the entire community.

Truth be told, I'm still not wild about walking or stair stepping, but as you can tell, I've tricked myself into enjoying it. Get creative and have a good time. You'll have some great stories to tell and it will help how you look and how you feel.

One more thing about walking. Is there anything else you could do while walking that will either be a good use of your time or maybe take the drudgery out of it for you? I've had my smartphone with me many times and have done e-mails, texting, answered calls, checked the weather, played games, made lists, set appointments, recorded ideas, and watched lap timing. I wouldn't suggest this stuff if you're not on a track. You may walk into a light pole or, worse yet, a car may run into you. Clearly, that won't help how you look or how you feel. Many walkers wear headphones or earbuds and listen to music or lectures or even watch TV shows. I get enough time under headphones at work so I don't do that, but it's an option for you.

Walking was the doctor's idea and it was a good one, but I've come up with many other ways to achieve the same thing. I'll share those with you next.

Chapter Seven

The "To Do" List

Some people aren't wild about "to do" lists, but I've always liked them because they improve my efficiency at getting things done. But now I have an even greater appreciation for the "to do" lists. Mine have helped me lose weight! If that's your goal, maybe this might work for you.

The only exercise the doctor mentioned was walking. Yes, that can be effective and it has been for me. As I mentioned, I've gotten a little creative with my walking, but you can get a lot more creative with your exercise beyond walking, and at the same time get some things done you've wanted to accomplish for a long time and burn calories while doing it.

What things have you wanted to get done but just don't seem to happen? Put them on a "to do" list. It's amazing how many things I had put off doing that turned out to be big calorie-burners. I discovered this the day I spent many hour long sessions transplanting plants from one part of my yard to another, where I really wanted them. I had put this off for a long time for two reasons. First, I knew it was going to be a huge job and that it would take several weeks to get it done. It seemed overwhelming. Secondly, because I was lazy. I almost hired someone to do it.

I put it on my to-do list where it stared me in the face until I finally got it done and checked it off. After the first day of doing it, I was sweaty and sore from the digging, hauling, watering and clean-up. I had planned to walk that evening, but it dawned on me that I had done more exercise and burned more calories transplanting than I would walking. So I skipped walking that day, wrote the transplanting down in my little book and counted the yardwork as my exercise.

During one follow-up appointment, the doctor was thumbing through my little book, saw the yardwork and said, "This is really good." I said, "Ya, but I didn't walk that day." He laughed and said, "That's fine. You got better exercise doing that than walking." I was glad that great minds thought alike! That to-do item did indeed last for nearly a month, as I worked on it a little at a time. I was thrilled to get it done and it was good for me. Plus I got to put that check mark by it on my list.

Garage-cleaning was on my list. I have two of them and they were both pig-sties. I sweated through both of those till I crossed them off the list. Again, there was great satisfaction in getting it done and using it as a way to exercise and burn calories. I love solving two problems by doing one thing!

Do you like to swim? I hadn't done it for a long time, so I put it on my to-do list. I looked into joining the YMCA so I could use their pool. They have wonderful facilities and staff but I found an alternative that cost less. I went to a local indoor aquatics center run by one of the cities in my area. The cost was four dollars to swim all day and only three dollars after six pm. Yes, you pay every time you swim, unless you get a yearly pass, but I only swim occasionally. If you want to do a lot of swimming, joining the Y would probably be wise, not to mention being able to use all their other equipment and services. Those would also help you burn calories. That, of course, assumes you actually go there and use them. I'm sure people that join fitness centers or buy fitness equipment have the highest intentions and hopes, but you really need to think through whether you will make good on a commitment to yourself to follow through, continually. We're only human, and evidence of that can be seen at garage sales with all the exercise gear and equipment for sale.

"Pull weeds!" That was another exercise on my list. In the past I had either ignored or mowed over them. The yard and the garden started looking better than it ever had. It was another way to get exercise and was another check mark on my list.

I've been to driving ranges, batting cages, bowling alleys, disc golf courses and other places I'd never visited before, all in the name of getting exercise and a workout. They have been, and will continue to be, on my list.

Pushups are on my list. I can't tell you how demoralized and discouraged I was when I first decided to try this. I was so overweight and so out of shape I could only do two of them! I have friends and relatives that can drop down and give you a hundred of them with seemingly little trouble. So, I thought about just dropping that idea, conceding I couldn't do it and forgetting the whole thing. It was demoralizing and humiliating for me.

Then I had an idea. What if I did pushups in such a way that every time I did them, I would do just one more than I did the last time? Even if I went from two to three pushups, that would be progress. I do both knee pushups and regular pushups and have astounded myself at the number of them I can now do. And the next time I do them, I will add one more. Pushups get a bit easier as you lose weight. You have less weight to lift. Chin-ups should be the same. I haven't mastered that. In fact, I find them even more discouraging than the pushups were, but dog-gone it, I'm gonna do it! Ironic isn't it that getting smaller can lead to personal growth if you do it properly?

And one last note about your To-Do list. Put it on the front of your refrigerator and the next time you go there to get something to eat, do one of your To-Do items instead!

Chapter Eight

The "Diet"

I've mentioned that people almost always gain weight when they go off a diet. My thought was that in taking on this project I needed to do it in such a way that there was no diet to end, thus having less chance to gain weight again.

So, instead of going on a diet I changed the way I ate forever! You hear dieticians, nutritionists and so-called weight-loss experts suggest this all the time, but it is often in one ear and out the other when you're not in the weight-loss mode. But I can tell you as a non-dietician, non-nutritionist average Joe, this is absolutely true! People on diets frequently have "goal weights," whether that's a number of pounds they want to lose or an actual weight they are targeting. I did not do that.

How do people celebrate accomplishment or achieving personal goals? Someone may say, "Congratulations! Let's go out and celebrate. You deserve a reward. You worked hard!" In your own mind, emotionally, you know you've done something good. It often kicks your thinking into an entirely different mindset. But how much sense does it make to switch from the mindset that brought you weight loss success? Not much. Many times those well intended, loving people that want to take you out to celebrate want to go where? A restaurant. You're a bit leery, but they tell you that you deserve it and it's time you rewarded yourself.

That's not a reward! That's a trigger! A trigger that can send you right back from where you came and to what you used to do. Be very, very careful! They were right. You worked hard for this. All the more reason not to invite trouble. It's not that you can't go to a restaurant and enjoy yourself. It's just that some restaurants either have nothing or very little that fits into your new lifestyle. Your friends will probably say something like, "Here, just have one bite of this cheesecake. One bite won't hurt you." That's a trigger! Don't pull it! It's a bit like trying to stop a fire by letting it die down, then, when you've had success, dumping some gas on it. Your well-meaning friends frequently will not understand what you've been through because they've never experienced it. When I've been out to eat with others, I've taken some chiding and even ridicule for being this way, but the big picture is much more important than that one moment.

So my weight-loss episode was not really a project, but a lifestyle change. If you're serious about this, I'd suggest that same change for you. Think about that from the beginning. You'll get plenty of rewards from the weight loss itself. After all, you want to look better and feel better, not starve yourself long enough that you "earn" more food that you probably shouldn't be eating anyway.

So, I guess you can have a goal weight if you think that would help you. It just wasn't something for me. When people tell me I look great, they often say, "Are you done now? And if not, how many more pounds are you going to lose?" My answer is "No," but I know that those asking are really asking if I'm done with my "diet". I'm not done with my diet because I was never on one. The "No" answer means "No. I'm not done with my new way of eating and never will be." The answer to the second part of their question is, "I don't know how many more pounds I will lose. I seldom even weigh myself. All I know is that I am eating healthy food of which the doctors and dieticians approve. When the weight-loss stops, it will stop. But my new way of life will not."

I'm a person of faith and I just feel that God knows better than I, or anyone else, what I should weigh. Just like every other area of my life, He's more of an expert than I'll ever be. That's a very liberating mindset, not only in weight-loss but in other areas of life as well.

So, with all that being said, I suggest that you do NOT go on a diet!

Chapter Nine

The Prescriptions

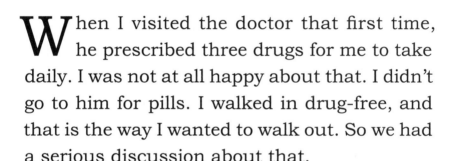

When I visited the doctor that first time, he prescribed three drugs for me to take daily. I was not at all happy about that. I didn't go to him for pills. I walked in drug-free, and that is the way I wanted to walk out. So we had a serious discussion about that.

He explained that I had one of the lowest levels of vitamin D that he had ever seen, that I was borderline diabetic and needed to lower my cholesterol and blood pressure and lose weight, thus the prescriptions. He had to do a lot of convincing to get me to take the drugs. I made clear to him that since I was the one that came to him and asked for help, I would do what he said, even though I knew about some of the down-sides of those particular drugs. I made sure that he knew my goal was to get back to being drug-free.

Our society has conditioned us to think a certain way when we hear the words "drug-free". The stereotype is of someone who was using illegal drugs, lost his/her home and family, went to a rehab program and is now "drug-free". Hallelujah for those situations, but by the numbers, those cases are dwarfed by people that take prescribed drugs, some-times many of them, every day. Those drugs have helped many people, but are often huge detriments to them as well. There is a reason that mandated disclaimers on commercials are read very quickly and at a lower enthu-siasm level, than the rest of the ad. Here are some disclaimers for no particular drug, but I know I have heard or seen each in various commercials:

Side effects may include vomiting, dizziness, death, darkened stool, depression, headache, dry mouth, thoughts of suicide, abdominal pain, and on and on.

Ya, doc! Give me some of that!!!

Nearly in the same breath, we are encouraged to ask our doctor if that drug is "right for you." Drug names are frequently hard to remember, but I suppose you could always ask the doctor if the one that would make you vomit and give you thoughts of suicide is right for you.

In another later visit to my doctor, he again went on and on about how disheartened he sometimes gets when patients, many at risk, listen to his advice, yet don't take it, and that I had done the opposite and really lifted his spirits. That made quite an impact on me. So much so that I picked up the phone and called the orthopedic surgeon, to whom I had originally told my bleak story and asked what he thought I should do. He was the one that got my foot in the door to see this particular doctor. I told him about all the good things that had happened to me since we spoke, including the massive weight- loss, and how grateful I was to him for being the catalyst to it all.

He said, "Wow!" There was a long pause, then these words, "You know, we doctors do this every day and we don't hear about dramatic results like yours. You are to be congratulated. You don't know how much your call means to me."

To be quite honest, I try to stay away from doctors, but these two guys had a tremendous effect on me. And it turns out I had a tremendous effect on them. That's very, very humbling.

By the way, after that last doctor's appointment, I went back to the office and my phone rang. It was his office. I'm a pretty positive person, but my initial thought was they found something else and something must be wrong. They called to tell me the doctor again reviewed my file. The message was, "You can now drop two of those prescriptions."

Bingo and Yippeee!!!

Chapter Ten

The Mindset

If I was going to change, I knew I absolutely had to draw a line in the sand in facing my unhealthy lifestyle. I had to admit it. I had to realize what I was doing to myself. I had to meet it head-on, honestly, and say, "That's it! Enough is enough! I'm going to meet this thing head-on and do something about it!" That's easier said than done, but you'll never get it done if you don't get it "said!" Again, if I continued to do what I'd already done, I'd continue to get what I'd already got, with the definition of insanity being doing the same thing and expecting different results.

So, if you are reading this because you truly do want to look better and feel better, I, from personal experience, ask you this question very directly....How badly do you really want this?

My guess is that since you picked up this book and are looking at it, your gut and your head are saying, "Yes, I really want to do this." Right now is the easiest time to answer that question. But what about tomorrow? What about the day after that? What about next week, next month, next year? I knew I had to have a hardcore commitment to this. It was fairly easy to say I would do it, but when you start your journey, you will immediately start walking through landmines. Some of those landmines are of your own making, but a lot of them come from sources over which you have absolutely no control.

Hunger pangs...what are you going to do about that?. What about other people in your life not wanting to eat what you need to eat, and their food and snacks are dangling there in front of you, free for the taking? What's your plan for that? How do you defend yourself when going out to restaurants?

Here's a monumental landmine for me, but I knew it was coming. For all ten days of the Iowa State Fair, I broadcast my radio show from a studio on the fairgrounds. Since food vendors know we are there and that we are well listened to, they bring in food, and a lot of it, to feed us, hoping we will mention it on the radio. I'm talking about corn dogs, ice cream, grinder Italian sandwiches, giant hot cinnamon rolls, lemonade, pork and beef sandwiches, pancakes, sausage and gravy, pizza, giant turkey drumsticks, tenderloins, funnel cakes...well, you get the idea. Our studio table was often not big enough for all the food!

I knew this was coming, so I had a plan. I turned it around and used it as motivation. If I could get through the Iowa State Fair without touching any of that, I figured I could get through anything! It seemed like the ultimate challenge. So I made it a goal. No matter how good it looked and smelled, and believe me, it looked and smelled fabulous, the goal was to touch none of it. If I could do that, it would be a giant victory for me, and could help me through the rest of my continual daily healthy living. During those days at the fair, the only thing I consumed while there was bottled water. That was quite a victory! Instead of feeling bloated, I had a feeling of pride and a feeling that, "Yes, I can do this!" I turned a negative into a positive.

Lesson....know that landmines are coming, and don't be shocked when they happen. Instead, be ready, having thought through this ahead of time. When the landmine comes, ask yourself again, "How badly do I really want to do this?" Since so many people have asked me, I'm glad to give advice, but in all honesty, if you don't have a bold, clear, strong, bull-headed answer to that question, you may be stuck with where you are, how you look and how you feel.

Frequently people are bull-headed about this for a week or a month, then the landmines are just too much for them. Not only is that demoralizing, they often wind up gaining back more weight than they lost because it turned out to be more of a diet than a way of life. By bull-headed I don't mean being obnoxious about it; just inwardly militant, while being outwardly polite!

Sometimes you may have to be honest and explain to people what you are doing and why you are doing it. Some will understand, or say they do, and be sympathetic right away. Others will be puzzled. Some will think you are nuts. Some probably will be inwardly thinking, "Ya, I bet that won't last long." That's all the more reason to make a super commitment to what you're doing and not only succeed, but make a huge impression on them in the future when they see the change in the way you look and the way you feel.

Chapter Eleven

The Food

I love grocery stores and always have. I see and use them differently now than I used to. I now spend most of my time in the produce department, whereas I used to spend a lot of that time at the Italian, Chinese, ice cream freezers, bakery and processed food aisles. I still spend just as much time as I used to at the store, and cover as much ground, but I now use the time strolling the aisles as walking time, not stopping very often unless two people are having a conversation and have the aisle blocked, or little Jimmy is having a fit in the cereal aisle. The grocery stores these days are big so you can do a lot of walking. The people that give out food samples on toothpicks stop me and compliment me on my new look and ask how I did it. Not being a smart aleck, I don't say, "By not eating what you're pushing." I'm not sure if they notice that I hardly ever take any of it, unless it's fruit or veggies. If I did, that would be a trigger...another one of those landmines.

Here is a more complete rundown of what I eat and when. After formerly eating no breakfast at all, I now have a bowl of oatmeal with raisins and walnuts after I get off the air at nine am. It probably doesn't make a lot of difference what kind of oatmeal it is, although I have plain, or what they call original, steel cut oatmeal. That sounds fancy, doesn't it? I have no idea what steel cut means, and I'm not so fascinated by it to dive into research, but you can bet they're not cutting this stuff with plastic silverware.

However, I would avoid all the foo-foo, shee-shee, flavored oatmeal out there. Usually they contain extra sugars and other things that are not what you want to be ingesting. I buy boxes of ten packets of steel cut oatmeal with flax. The one I buy is labeled "classic", and all the other boxes around it have all the extra flavor additives. Each one of the packets is easy to use, because you simply cut the top off, dump the oatmeal into a cup, add a couple of spoonsful of raisins and walnuts, then fill the empty oatmeal pouch with water, pour the water in the cup, and microwave. At home, it only takes two-and-a-half minutes. At work, we apparently have a cheapo microwave because it takes three-and-a-half there.

Do you have to put raisins in it? No. You don't have to add fruit if you don't want it, but I have also used fresh strawberries, blueberries, and/or peaches. Do you have to put walnuts in?. No. I like the extra crunch, and walnuts are one of the more nutritious nuts. You can use other nuts or none at all. I get the nuts in bags in the baking aisle. At first, I was shocked to see that these bags of nuts are very expensive. On the other hand, I'm saving so much money by not buying a lot of the bad stuff I used to buy that I'm still saving money. If you eat your oatmeal plain, that's fine, but I find it a bit bland and the fruit will sweeten it up a little. That's my breakfast.

Now lunch...It's very simple. I have one six ounce serving of yogurt, which is the container size most companies sell. I buy ten at a time in different flavors. People always want to know whether to get Greek or regular. I frequently hear that Greek is better for you, but I'm not convinced. However there is an argument that it often has less sugar. Some do. Many people like the thickness of the Greek. I like the regular, but the Greek is growing on me. Do watch out for yogurts with candies, sweet flavorings, chocolate and artificial additives. It doesn't make much sense to get candy bar-flavored yogurt, given what you are trying to achieve. Seems to me that is a bit like washing sleeping pills down with coffee.

When the doctor mentioned the yogurt, I asked him about the fact that I knew it had sugar. He said it was so small that I shouldn't worry about it, so I don't. For the most part, that's about the only processed sugar I eat. But as time goes on I'm opting for yogurt with less or no sugar or sweeteners in it. I put in some fruit. I've enjoyed it, even though I've never really been a big yogurt fan before this, and it seems to be effective. When I get home from the store with the yogurt, I put them in the fridge, then grab one the next morning to take to work. I purposely don't look at the flavor, so I get a fun surprise when I pull it out of the fridge at work at noon. As I mentioned earlier, that's really rather pathetic isn't it? That's what life has come to!

Now dinner...Pretty simple as well, but it gives you a chance for a bit more variety and creativity. Basically, it is one piece of lean meat, a vegetable and fruit for dessert. The easiest tasty meat for me to prepare is boneless, skinless chicken breast. Portion control is easy when you have one or two, if they're small. I have purchased fresh, never frozen, but I also have purchased breasts frozen, with eight to twelve per bag. As far as preparation, I think I have done everything a person could possibly do to a chicken.... grilled, steamed, baked, air-fried, microwaved, shredded, slow-cooked, stir-fried and more. I even tried grilling the frozen chicken straight out of the bag and it made the end result surprisingly juicy.

Not only are there many ways you can prepare this part of the meal, there are several other meats you can use for the same thing. Turkey is similar and low in fat. An occasional beef or pork item is fine and fish is a great item as well. As a side note, if you grill fish, oil up the grill grate very well before you put on the fish.

Fish is so low in fat it will stick to the grill and make a mess, and you may even lose part of it into the grill. I speak from experience, but I've learned and don't have that problem anymore.

As far as the vegetables go, choose what you like, but colorful veggies will serve you better. I mentioned to a kid one time that colorful foods were better for you. He said, "Good, I eat Cheetos." Shoot for naturally colorful, not chemically. Broccoli, beets, carrots, asparagus, you decide. I usually steam them, and you can even buy them in microwave steamer bags. I've grilled some, but usually on foil with some oil. One thing I've enjoyed is buying lettuce or collard greens with the largest leaves I can find. Sometimes I'll make a chicken sandwich using the leaves as a wrap rather than bread. I know of one deli sandwich chain that will do the same for you.

This brings up an interesting point. I have had no bread since that first doctor's appointment. That was hard for me, because I've always loved burgers, sandwiches, pizza, and almost all bready things. That was part of my problem. Bread has not been good to me, especially with its processed white flour and extra additives like preservatives. I noticed on some bread packages they brag about adding vitamins or minerals or whatever. That's because any of those that were in it originally were frequently processed out in the first place.

So, between not eating bread and sugars, except in the yogurt, that pretty much leaves out cookies, cakes, donuts, pies, rolls, and many other "staples" of the American diet that have made us fat. I haven't had ice cream for a long time. For after dinner dessert I have come to love small frozen fruits in a bowl with some nuts mixed in. The fruit doesn't need to be frozen, but I like it that way. One of my favorites is frozen bananas. I buy a bunch, peel them, cut them in half and put them in cheapo sandwich bags, one per bag. To me they taste like banana ice cream.

Then there is one other thing that I seldom eat, and it pains me to talk about this because it is one of my favorite foods in the world. Cheese! I love cheese! Yet I've had very little for a long, long time. It's not that cheese is so bad.....it's just that I would be like an alcoholic with it. One bite and I would want more...and more...and more. Another trigger! So Van, (or fill in your name here), how badly do you really want to do this? Are you willing to give up a few favorites? Maybe your very favorite? There will be a food or foods that will be a real test for you too. You may agonize over it, but the longer you don't eat it, the easier it gets to resist. These things are the real test of your commitment of how badly you really want to do this. That's good, not bad. Think of that ahead of time and be prepared psychologically, because it's coming! You have been warned!

So there you have it...the details of breakfast, lunch and dinner, along with some warnings that will help you, if you really, truly want it to create amazing results in how you look and how you feel!

Chapter Twelve

The Specialists

After that first doctor's visit, he set up tests from cardiologists, blood specialists, pulmonologists, endocrinologists, urologists, hematologists, gastroenterologists....let's put it this way....if their title had "gist" on the end, I saw them and they saw me. To be honest, I felt like running away that month. Here I am, a guy that never goes to see a doctor and now I'm seeing all of them! It wasn't easy getting appointments with these people and getting through the appointments was no fun.

One of these appointments was so far down the calendar that I had actually lost quite a bit of weight by then. As fate would have it, this specialist was a friend of mine that I hadn't seen for a long time. He's a great guy and I consider him a good friend. Oddly enough, he is overweight. In fact, as bad as I was, he was bigger and has been ever since I've known him. When he walked into the exam room, he said, "Wow! You've lost a lot of weight!" (Since that day, I have lost double that amount.) He said, "I really need to do that too."

He quizzed me about my situation and did a few tests. After that he said, "I don't know what you're doing, but you're doing all the right things. Now we need to put you through some more detailed tests. That's what I do you know. That's my job." He was a bit defensive about it. He probably could tell I was a bit disgusted. He didn't say so, but I got the impression he didn't really think they were necessary but that he should do them anyway.

I gambled, maybe because he was my friend, and said, "Well, if you give a guy a hammer, he's gonna go around looking for nails." Luckily he laughed hard. So he said, "Ya, you're right. I'll tell you what...let's make an appointment for a year from now and we'll see if you've been able to keep up this progress or if we should dive into this further." I told him I thought that was a great idea.

Then we had what I thought was a startling discussion. I told him about the medications the doctor had prescribed for me and that I wanted to get off of them. He looked at my chart to see what they were. One of them was a drug he himself was taking. He named it, said it was an amazing drug and that he thought everyone should be taking it. "Don't you agree?" he said. I snapped, "No! I'd like to see as many people as possible off as many drugs as possible and leading a life that leads to as few pills as possible!" He agreed, but said how fortunate we are to have drugs like these.

On my way home I was troubled by that conversation and thought about it deeply, trying to understand why he would think everyone should be on that drug. I'm no doctor, pharmacist, or scientist but I came to the conclusion that the drug he was talking about was one he was taking because of what his overweight situation was doing to him, and that the drug, as opposed to all the types of changes I'd been making, was keeping him alive.

I did not go back a year later. I had lost fifty more pounds and didn't feel it necessary. Perhaps I should have......for his sake. One day he will probably read this, and even though I have not named him, his practice or even his area of expertise, he'll know I'm talking about him. I pray he won't be offended. But at this point, I'm just trying to do the same thing I know he wants to do....help people.

Chapter Thirteen

The Results

If you want to change, what results are you looking for? I got the results I wanted. I no longer fall asleep at my desk. I don't sweat or get winded doing ordinary things. At three in the morning, when the alarm goes off, it is still a shock even after all those years of doing it, but once I gain consciousness, I'm up and on my way. As I mentioned, there was a time when I didn't think I could do it anymore. It is astounding how much better I now feel at that time of morning which, in actuality, is still the middle of the night for most people, me included. In fact I feel better all the time. I'm even OK with looking at myself in the mirror. I used to hate that, so I didn't often do it. And I hate looking at pictures of myself before I changed. Here are a few. You look at them. I can't stand to.

BEFORE

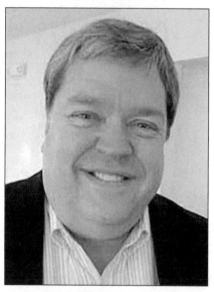

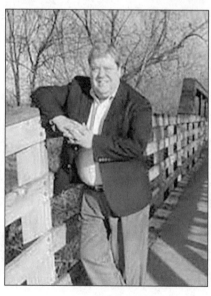

In short, I now look better and feel better. And here are some "after" pictures that I can look at without wincing. By the way, I know the one with Superman and me together is confusing since we're never seen together at the same time, so just for clarity, that's me on the left.

AFTER

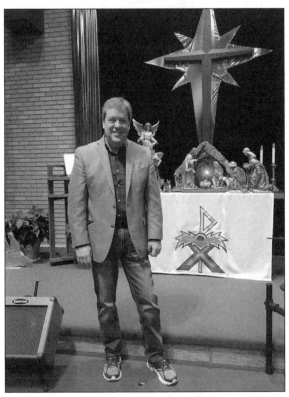

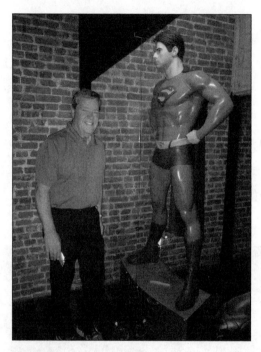

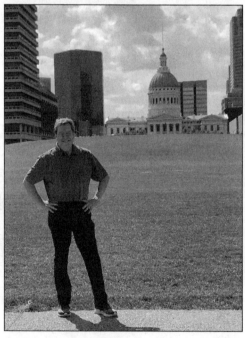

What results do YOU want? If you haven't thought about that, do it! It is said that many people have no goal and are hitting the target with one hundred percent accuracy. No one gets in a car, bus, plane or train without knowing where he/she wants to go. It doesn't necessarily have to be a specific weight, but if your goal is to improve the way you look and the way you feel, I've done the best I can to tell you what worked for me. Will it work for you? I don't know, but if you really, truly want this, are bull headed about it, stay consistent and let minor setbacks bounce off you, I'm convinced the answer is YES! In fact, if all those are true, I don't see how it could NOT have an awesome, perhaps life-changing effect on you.

One result of which you should be aware is that people will pay more attention and be more attracted to you. Are you ready for that? I'm serious! Are you ready for people to treat you differently than they used to, even though you are the same person? I know what you're saying... "Absolutely! Bring it on!". Maybe that's the result you're looking for. Be ready and be careful, especially if you are married. Make a recommitment to your spouse before you even start this. It's flattering to get "hit on," especially if it has been a long time since it has happened, or maybe it never has.

I am writing this warning to you as though you have already tried what I have done, were successful at it, look better and feel better. That's getting the cart way before the horse, but it's very important to think about. When it happens, you'll know it in a moment, and it will be good that you thought about it ahead of time. It's a tremendous thing to look and feel better, but if you aren't ready for the results, or mismanage them, you could actually cause a lot of damage not just for you, but for others. If you decide to do these things I have written, do them for the right reasons. If you do, it will serve you well!

A final result will be the personal satisfaction of knowing there was something you wanted, you made a plan for it to happen, you stuck to your guns and it worked! There is only one person on the face of this earth that will determine if this will work or not. That's you! A million doctors, personal trainers, diet plans, exercise machines, psychologists, counselors or fitness centers are not going to help you if you are not driving this new lifestyle yourself. That's why I only used one of them, the doctor. I am happily seeing less and less of him and have shed most of the prescriptions, making good, at least partially, on that vow to get rid of him and the drugs. I am indeed very grateful to him for jump-starting me to do this on my own.

Chapter Fourteen

The Loved Ones

M any of you are reading this for your own sake, or perhaps your real concern is for someone you love or care about. As you read the things in this book you may be thinking, "Yes, yes, yes!" But how in the world do you get someone else interested in it? I remember being in church and hearing a few messages, thinking, "Wow, I wish so-and-so was here listening to this."

When I was large, I didn't like people bringing up my size and my health, even when they were doing it because they cared about me and were concerned. I knew the situation full well and wasn't happy with it either. But it was more frustrating than helpful to hear anyone else bringing it up. In fact it almost made me more rebellious. You just want the whole issue to go away. Well, if you die, it will! That's what's so concerning to you if you are a loved one worrying about someone who is not healthy. I have had several friends and co-workers that were overweight, yet younger than I, that died of heart attacks. I miss them dearly.

Since my change, I have had a lot of radio listeners telling me how concerned they were about me before I changed and how thankful they were that I addressed the issue. Through the years, I've done many TV commercials, have made thousands of public appearances, and have had my picture on billboards, newspapers, magazines and social media. It used to be that you could be in the radio business and hide your appearance but we're way beyond that now.

I've had listeners hug me and cry and say, "You've got to help me! I'm so worried about my spouse." Which leads back to the question, how do you get someone you really care about to make a change? Given my own experience, here is what I would suggest: Mention it to him/her ONCE in the most loving way you can. ONCE! Make sure you make it clear that it was your heart that lead you to say it simply because of how much you care about him/her. Tell them you'll never, ever mention it again. Believe me, that moment will be hot-branded into their memory. Saying anything more about it after that is totally unnecessary, counterproductive and like rubbing salt in the wound or heaping more coals on an already large fire. If someone would have harped at me over and over, I would have resented it and it would have had exactly the opposite of the intended effect.

So, will the "one-and-done" method work? Some may respond quickly. Some will respond in their own time after they process it for themselves. That could be a week or ten years. Some will never respond, but that's not your fault. You will have done everything you should and could do to help. You're going to worry about them, but never ever think you didn't do enough. Some things are out of your control. Pray for them and go in peace with that.

Chapter Fifteen

The Emotions

C learly there are a lot of physical and bio-
logical things going on when you try to
look better and feel better. Exercise and nutri-
ents are all about biology and physiology. But
there's something that is at least that important,
if not more so. That is your state of mind, your
attitude, your emotions and your perception. A
lot of this, to be quite honest, is a head game.
It can propel you to success, or plummet you
to failure.

Most of what I've said here in this book probably sounds pretty good on paper and hopefully
is encouraging to you. If you've ever made a
New Year's resolution, started a diet or planted
a garden, you know what a good feeling it is in
the beginning having a plan, a commitment and

great intentions. Those are all critical steps, but then the real "fun" begins....actually doing it.

I suggest keeping this book nearby after you're done reading it, then rereading it, or at least the parts of it that most resonate with you, frequently, even when things are going well. It will be especially important when you disappoint yourself, or get down about not doing as well as you'd like. Actually, it's absolutely critical that you have moments like that! That may sound odd, but until you conquer, or at least make it through, moments like that, you probably can't reach your objective. You're going to have to go through these things and learn from them to make this thing work.

Sometimes when you disappoint yourself, you may think something is terribly wrong and get disgusted or even quit. Let me talk you off the ledge right now. These things are going to happen! Period! Expect them. Don't be surprised. Use them in a positive way. What did you learn from it? Save that for the future. What does a boxer do when he gets punched to the mat? They all do, by the way. He has two choices...lay there with bruises, including his ego, in disgust...or learn from it, get up, bruises and all, and get back to doing exactly what he knows he should do. I just want to encourage you when those moments come, and they will. Don't think to yourself "This doesn't work," and give up. Setbacks are an important part of how it DOES work!

There also is the opposite emotion. Some people have success and get cocky. That won't work, at least not for long. When you have success, be grateful for what has happened, keep doing what you're doing and get your mind off yourself. Celebrate success by going out and helping other people that need help.....at anything! I said in the beginning, and I'll say it again, generally speaking, people spend too much time thinking about themselves, me included.

Chapter Sixteen

The Thing to Drink

I've been thinking back to what I may have left out for you. I told you about food and exercise, but I didn't mention what you should drink. I've heard that about sixty percent of your body is water. Blood is about ninety-two percent water. The brain is about seventy-five percent water, and even bones are twenty-two percent water. Now, you tell me.. what should you drink?

I love fruit juice and when I was large, I drank a lot of it often. After all, fruit is healthy and we're supposed to get plenty of that, right? When I proudly told the doctor I drank lots of fruit juice, instead of getting an "Atta boy!" he said without hesitation, "Stop doing that. Too much sugar." Right or wrong, just about the only thing I drink now is water. Occasionally

I will have some pure carrot or beet juice and I might have a small glass of wine on a special occasion, but rarely. There are some pretty good, flavored sparkling waters on the market, but read those labels carefully. If it has sugar, sugar substitute, or other additives, forget it.

As a matter of fact that's a good rule for anything canned or packaged, whether it is food or drink. For a while, I studied and tried to learn about all the bad ingredients they put in things these days so I could read the labels and avoid them, but I found it exhausting, demoralizing and infuriating. So I came up with my own simple rule. If there are over four ingredients listed, don't buy it. Simple as that.

For some people, drinking water almost exclusively is easy to do. I fall into that category. Other people may have to grin and bear it. At least it doesn't have a bad taste! I constantly see people carrying cases of pop out of the grocery store. That's fruit juice on steroids. Don't drink it. So, there....the topic of what to drink has been covered.

Chapter Seventeen

The Setbacks and Disappointments

—◇✕◇—

I'm going to spend more time on this with you because you'll have them....guaranteed. It can be frustrating, demoralizing, disgusting, discouraging and make you feel like a failure. There is good news and bad news about that. The good news....you know you slipped up and didn't live up to your commitment to yourself. The bad news....it could lead you to lose your momentum, or even quit! Here you are trying so hard to do all the right things. Then you'll eat something you shouldn't have eaten. You'll skip some exercising. You'll eat more than you should have. You may get discouraged or mad at yourself.

We've already determined it's not a matter of IF it happens, because it will. The real question is how are you going to handle it when it does? Well, as with a lot of things in life, you either get bitter or you get better! Bitterness helps no one, especially you. But learning from the experience and using that insight for the future is of huge value...if you use it that way.

When I was a kid I grew up on a golf course, so my parents put a club in my hand as soon as I could hold one. I got pretty good at it, being both on my high school and college teams. I learned a lot about life from golf. When I hit a bad shot and it went down into the ditch, it made me mad! The madder I was, the worse the next shot was. But when I took each one a shot at a time, whether I was in the ditch or the middle of the fairway, and put the past behind, which really didn't matter anymore, the better I did with the next shot. There were a number of times that I shot a ball out of the ditch and it landed on the green. I putted it in and it was like I had never been in the ditch at all! I've seen other golfers in the ditch swearing and even throwing clubs. It always got worse for them. You get the point. If you goof up, life gives you the opportunity to redeem yourself, unless you'd rather sit around, have a pity party, get mad or beat yourself up. That never ever makes things better.

So, be prepared, and learn from mistakes and disappointments. When you look back, you'll be glad you did. In fact you may even be glad you had those disappointments and realize they helped you get where you were going!

Chapter Eighteen

The End

So, my conscience feels better now. I needed to write this before I died for two reasons.... one: Maybe it will help someone....and two: It's difficult to write a book AFTER you die. I wrote it by popular demand after being bombarded with questions and requests. When I've met people that have sought me out, a lot of the guys pat their bellies three times and say, "Ya, I need to get rid of this." I don't know why it's three times, but I swear it always is. Some people, men and women, have told me they had just a few pounds they needed to shed. Others, like I did, have a considerable number of pounds to lose.

All of us can clearly see what an epidemic this is by merely looking around at others, but it seems that more people are thinking about it more deeply and want to do something about their situation. Like you maybe? After all, you're reading this book. My heart, thoughts and prayers are with you and your loved ones in your journey of improving the way you look and the way you feel. I hope something within these pages will help.